Optimal Fitness

From Exercise to Recovery

by Bruce Goldwell

Health Disclaimer:

The information provided in this book is intended for general educational and informational purposes only. It is not a substitute for professional medical advice, diagnosis, or treatment. Always seek the advice of a qualified healthcare provider or physician with any questions you may have regarding your health or a medical condition. Never disregard professional medical advice or delay in seeking it because of something you have read in this book. The author, publisher, and contributors of this book are not healthcare professionals, and the content presented here should not be considered as a replacement for professional medical guidance. The information provided should be used in conjunction with the expertise and guidance of a healthcare professional. Individual responses to health strategies and recommendations may vary. It is essential to consult with a healthcare provider before making any significant changes to your diet, exercise routine, or healthcare management plan. The author and publisher do not assume any liability for any direct, indirect, or consequential damage or injury resulting from the use or misinterpretation of the information provided in this book. Readers are encouraged to consult with their healthcare providers for personalized advice and to ensure that any recommendations or strategies discussed in this book are safe and appropriate for their specific health conditions and circumstances.

Preface

At the height of his weight gain, Bruce tipped the scales at 215 pounds. Upon realizing he had gradually let himself deteriorate and exceed his ideal weight, he took action. His weight loss journey commenced slowly and in a piecemeal fashion. Despite the struggles, Bruce eventually managed to weigh less than 200 pounds. He would adopt a technique, lose about five pounds, plateau, and then abandon the approach. Eventually, following contemporary exercise plans allowed him to shed an additional five pounds at a time. Gradually over the years, Bruce reached weights below 180 pounds.

Once he maintained a weight of 175 for several years, he decided it was time to get serious about his weight loss journey. He embarked on research to discover more structured methods for losing weight. Eager to share his knowledge and assist others in similar situations, Bruce authored a book outlining some of what he learned. Currently, Bruce weighs 160 pounds thanks to intermittent fasting and carefully selected supplements that support his body management lifestyle. He is now accelerating the process of loosing weight and building back his muscle strength and inductance.

This eBook is now the latest of his findings which focuses on recovery and ways to help if not accelerate the process. This should only be the beginning of your process of learning about your body, how it functions internally, and how you can best capitalize on your own body management lifestyle.

Be sure to read all the way through. Don't worry if you don't absorb all the information in one read. To insure you have gained as much insight as needed to change the things you need to in your workout regimen, read as many times as needed to absorb the content. Take notes of those things you find most important. Links are included to supplements that the author has researched and determined to best support building stronger muscles and aiding in the recovery process.

Your feedback is invaluable in improving my authorship.

(Your support helps me support other vets too.)

As a Vietnam Veteran, I strive to assist my fellow Vets whenever possible. Homeless veterans face daily challenges in obtaining basic necessities like food. To enhance my ability to help more veterans, I kindly request your support. *By reviewing my books and sharing them with others,* my fan base can grow, allowing for increased readership. With a larger audience, my royalties will increase, providing me with the resources to financially support not only veterans but also anyone needing assistance. **Thank you for your support.**

Table of Contents

Optimal Fitness

From Exercise to Recovery

Nourishing Your Journey

The Importance of a Balanced Diet

Welcome to "Optimal Fitness: From Exercise to Recovery." This book aims to provide comprehensive guidance on maintaining muscle mass, recovering from workouts, and cultivating a truly healthy lifestyle. Before embarking on this journey, it is essential to establish an understanding of the human body and its critical functions in relation to fitness and well-being.

Our journey begins by examining the importance of a balanced diet. Nutrition plays a pivotal role in muscle growth, fueling workouts, and supporting overall health. As you progress through the chapter, you will learn about the physiological processes that allow for muscle growth, such as protein synthesis and muscle fiber adaptation. Emphasis will be placed on whole foods, adequate hydration, and macro-nutrient balance for optimal results.

Next, we will delve into how various forms of exercise contribute to maintaining muscle mass. Topics will include resistance training, cardiovascular workouts, and flexibility routines – all crucial components of any fitness plan. We will discuss evidence-based approaches for different exercises and offer practical tips for incorporating them into your weekly routine.

Determining one's optimal caloric intake is often a challenge. In this chapter, guidance will be provided on calculating daily calorie needs and achieving an ideal balance of carbohydrates, proteins, and fats tailored to your unique goals and lifestyle.

Exercise selection is paramount in building muscle effectively. The chapter provides an overview of various workout techniques that promote muscle growth by stimulating different muscle groups. You will be introduced to specific exercises for beginning or advancing your strength training journey.

A crucial component in any successful fitness plan is appropriately scheduling workouts to avoid over-training while ensuring sufficient recovery time. We will discuss workout frequency, rest periods, and the importance of including rest days in your routine.

Preventing over-training comes hand in hand with understanding the signs of overexertion on the body. We provide information on recognizing symptoms like fatigue or decreased performance and strategies for avoiding potential risks.

The chapter will further explore the vital processes of muscle repair, glycogen replenishment, and the impact of sleep on recovery. As you delve deeper into these topics, you will come to appreciate the importance of quality rest, stress management, and good sleep hygiene for overall health.

As our population ages, the natural decline in muscle mass becomes increasingly relevant. The chapter addresses this concern by discussing strategies to counteract age-related muscle loss through targeted exercise and thoughtful nutrition choices.

Hormones play a fundamental role in muscle growth and maintenance. We will discuss hormonal influence on muscle development, primarily focusing on testosterone, growth hormone, and insulin.

We also shed light upon extreme diets and supplements which might promise quick gains but come with health hazards. Instead, we emphasize a balanced approach as a foundation for sustainable progress.

Measuring progress is essential to stay motivated in any fitness journey. The chapter provides guidance on goal setting, progress tracking and using various metrics like body composition to

chart your path forward effectively.
Lastly, psychological aspects also play an essential role in maintaining muscle mass and staying committed to one's fitness goals. The importance of motivation, discipline and mental well-being will be highlighted throughout the chapter.

In conclusion, this first chapter lays the groundwork for your journey towards sustainable health, vitality, and muscular fitness. By understanding the fundamentals outlined here – from nutrition to recovery – you will be well-equipped to make informed decisions that lead to long-term success in your fitness endeavors. Let us begin our journey together towards optimal health and peak performance.

Foundations of Fitness

Understanding Your Body and Health

Understanding the human body and how it functions is crucial for overall health and fitness. Here are some important questions that should be answered to help people know more about their bodies and how to maintain proper muscle mass, recover from workouts, and stay healthy:

1. What is the importance of a balanced diet?
   - Understanding the role of nutrition in maintaining overall health, supporting muscle growth, and fueling workouts.

2. How does the body build and maintain muscle mass?
   - Explaining the physiological processes involved in muscle growth, including protein synthesis and muscle fiber adaptation.

3. What is the significance of exercise in maintaining muscle mass?
   - Clarifying the role of resistance training, cardiovascular exercise, and flexibility routines in preserving and increasing muscle mass.

4. How can individuals determine their optimal caloric intake and macro-nutrient ratios?
   - Providing guidance on how to calculate daily

calorie needs and the ideal balance of carbohydrates, proteins, and fats.

5. What are the best exercises for muscle building?
   - Discussing various resistance training techniques, exercises, and workout programs that promote muscle growth.

6. How often should people work out to maintain muscle mass?
   - Explaining the importance of workout frequency, recovery periods, and rest days in muscle-building routines.

7. What are the signs of over-training, and how can they be prevented?
   - Informing individuals about the risks of excessive exercise, signs of over-training, and strategies for avoiding it.

8. How does the body recover from workouts?
   - Discussing the processes of muscle repair, glycogen replenishment, and the role of sleep in recovery.

9. What is the impact of sleep and rest on muscle recovery and overall health?
   - Highlighting the importance of quality sleep, rest, and stress management for optimal recovery and muscle growth.

10. How can individuals manage and prevent workout-related injuries?

   - Providing information on injury prevention strategies, proper warm-ups, cool-downs, and form during exercises.

11. What are the effects of aging on muscle mass and how can it be mitigated?

   - Discussing the natural decline in muscle mass and strength with age and strategies to counteract this through exercise and nutrition.

12. What role do hormones play in muscle growth and maintenance?

   - Explaining the influence of hormones like testosterone, growth hormone, and insulin in muscle development.

13. What are the health risks of extreme diets and supplements for muscle growth?

   - Discussing the potential dangers of extreme dieting, excessive supplementation, and the importance of a balanced approach.

14. How can individuals set and track fitness goals?

   - Providing guidance on goal setting, progress tracking, and the use of metrics like body composition measurements.

15. What are the psychological aspects of

maintaining muscle mass and fitness?
   - Addressing the importance of motivation, discipline, and mental well-being in achieving and sustaining fitness goals.

Answering these questions can help individuals make informed decisions about their fitness and overall health, enabling them to create effective and sustainable plans for muscle maintenance, recovery, and well-being.

What is the importance of a balanced diet?

The importance of a balanced diet cannot be overstated when it comes to maintaining overall health, supporting muscle growth, and fueling workouts. A balanced diet is crucial because it provides the necessary nutrients and energy your body needs for various functions, including muscle growth and exercise performance. Let's break down the significance of a balanced diet in more detail:

1. Nutrient Intake: A balanced diet ensures that you receive a wide variety of essential nutrients, including vitamins, minerals, carbohydrates, proteins, and fats. These nutrients are essential for the proper functioning of the body. For example:

   - **Carbohydrates** are your body's primary source of energy. They provide the fuel necessary for daily activities and workouts.

   - **Proteins** are the building blocks of muscle tissue. Adequate protein intake is crucial for muscle repair and growth, making it essential for those looking to increase or maintain muscle mass.

   - **Vitamins and minerals** are involved in numerous metabolic processes, supporting overall health and helping your body function optimally.

2. Energy Balance: To maintain a healthy body weight and support muscle growth or exercise performance, it's important to maintain an appropriate energy balance. A balanced diet helps you control your calorie intake and expenditure, which is essential for weight management. Consuming more calories than you burn can lead to weight gain, while consuming fewer calories can lead to weight loss. A balanced diet allows you to meet your energy needs without overeating or under-eating.

3. Muscle Growth: As mentioned, proteins are critical for muscle growth. A balanced diet provides an adequate supply of protein, enabling your body to repair and build new muscle tissue. This is especially important for individuals engaging in resistance training and strength exercises. Without a balanced diet, you might not get the necessary amino acids and protein intake to support muscle development.

4. Exercise Performance: To fuel your workouts and maximize performance, you need the right balance of macro-nutrients and micro-nutrients Carbohydrates provide energy for high-intensity activities, while fats play a role in sustained, lower-intensity exercise. Consuming a variety of nutrients ensures that you have the stamina and strength needed for workouts. Inadequate nutrition can lead to fatigue, decreased exercise performance, and impaired recovery. (See Support Products Page.)

5. Overall Health: A balanced diet contributes to overall health by reducing the risk of chronic diseases, promoting cardiovascular health, and supporting a strong immune system. Nutrient-rich foods help protect against illnesses and maintain vitality.

6. Weight Management: For those interested in maintaining or achieving a healthy body weight, a balanced diet helps in controlling calorie intake, managing hunger, and preventing overeating. It also reduces the risk of weight-related health issues.

A balanced diet is essential for overall health, muscle growth, and exercise performance. It ensures that your body receives the right combination of nutrients and energy to function optimally, repair and build muscle, and sustain workouts. By understanding the role of nutrition in these aspects, individuals can make informed dietary choices that support their fitness and health goals.

How does the body build and maintain muscle mass?

Building and maintaining muscle mass involves complex physiological processes. Understanding these processes is crucial for anyone looking to optimize their muscle growth and preserve their hard-earned gains. Two key factors in this context are protein synthesis and muscle fiber adaptation. Here's a detailed explanation of how the body builds and maintains muscle mass:

1. Protein Synthesis:

a. Muscle Protein Synthesis (MPS): Muscle growth, also known as hypertrophy, occurs primarily through a process called muscle protein synthesis. MPS is the creation of new muscle proteins, particularly myofibrillar proteins, which make up the contractile units of muscle fibers.

b. Stimulus for MPS: Muscle growth is initiated in response to mechanical stress or resistance, typically during strength training or resistance exercises. When you lift weights or perform resistance exercises, you create microscopic damage to muscle fibers. This damage is a signal to your body to repair and remodel the muscle tissue.

c. Nutrient Involvement: Adequate protein intake is critical for muscle protein synthesis. After a workout, especially resistance training, your body becomes more sensitive to dietary protein. Consuming protein-rich foods or supplements post-workout provides the amino acids needed for repairing and building muscle tissue.

d. Role of Amino Acids: Amino acids, the building blocks of protein, are essential for MPS. Among the amino acids, leucine plays a significant role as a signaling molecule that activates protein synthesis pathways.

e. Timing: Timing is important. Consuming protein shortly after a workout maximizes the anabolic (muscle-building) response. The post-workout window is often referred to as the "anabolic window."

2. Muscle Fiber Adaptation:

a. Muscle Fiber Types: The human body has different types of muscle fibers, broadly categorized as Type I (slow-twitch) and Type II (fast-twitch) fibers. Type II fibers are further subdivided into Type IIa and Type IIb (or IIx).

b. Training Adaptation: Resistance training stimulates muscle fiber adaptation. The extent to which a muscle fiber grows or strengthens depends on factors like the intensity of the training, the load lifted, and the number of repetitions performed.

c. Hypertrophy: Muscle hypertrophy can result from both increased muscle fiber size and an increase in the number of contractile proteins within the fibers. The size of muscle fibers can increase due to an increase in the number and size of myofibrils within the fiber.

d. Neural Adaptation: Initially, strength gains in resistance training are often attributed to neural adaptation. This means your body becomes more efficient at recruiting muscle fibers to perform a given task. Over time, actual muscle hypertrophy contributes significantly to strength gains.

3. Recovery and Rest:

a. Rest and Repair: The growth and repair of muscle tissue occur during rest and recovery periods, not during the workout itself. It's essential to provide your body with adequate sleep and recovery time to allow these processes to take place.

b. Nutrition and Hydration: Proper nutrition, including adequate protein intake and hydration, supports muscle repair and adaptation. Micro-nutrients like vitamins and minerals also play roles in various metabolic processes related to muscle growth.

Building and maintaining muscle mass is a dynamic process involving muscle protein synthesis, muscle fiber adaptation, and appropriate recovery. Strength training or resistance exercises serve as the stimulus for muscle growth, while proper nutrition and rest are essential for optimizing the process. Understanding these physiological processes can help individuals tailor their workouts, nutrition, and recovery strategies to achieve their muscle-building goals effectively.

What is the significance of exercise in maintaining muscle mass?

Exercise plays a pivotal role in maintaining and increasing muscle mass. To understand the significance of exercise in this context, we need to clarify the specific roles that different types of exercises, including resistance training, cardiovascular exercise, and flexibility routines, play in preserving and promoting muscle mass:

1. Resistance Training:

- **Muscle Stimulation:** Resistance training, often involving lifting weights or using resistance bands, is the primary form of exercise that directly stimulates muscle growth. It places stress on muscle fibers, creating tiny micro-tears in the muscle tissue. The body then repairs and rebuilds these tears, resulting in increased muscle size and strength.

- **Hypertrophy:** Resistance training promotes muscle hypertrophy, which is the process of muscle fibers growing in size. It particularly targets the fast-twitch muscle fibers, which have a higher potential for hypertrophy.

- **Metabolic Benefits:** Resistance training boosts metabolism, as muscle tissue is more metabolically active than fat tissue. This means that individuals with a higher percentage of lean muscle mass burn more calories at rest, which can be beneficial for weight management.

- **Functional Strength:** Resistance training enhances functional strength, making daily activities easier and reducing the risk of injury. It's also crucial for athletes and individuals interested in sports performance.

- **Bone Health:** Resistance training has secondary benefits for bone health. It can help increase bone density, which is particularly important as people age to reduce the risk of osteoporosis.

2. Cardiovascular Exercise:

- **Supporting Overall Health:** Cardiovascular exercise, such as running, swimming, or cycling, is essential for overall health. While it doesn't directly stimulate muscle growth in the same way as resistance training, it helps improve circulation, heart health, and lung capacity.

- **Calorie Burn:** Cardiovascular exercise can assist in weight management by burning calories. It's a valuable addition to a balanced fitness routine when combined with resistance training, as it helps create a calorie deficit if weight loss is a goal.

- Endurance and Stamina: Cardiovascular exercise enhances endurance and stamina, which can support more productive and efficient resistance training sessions.

3. Flexibility Routines:

- Injury Prevention: Maintaining flexibility is crucial for injury prevention. Stretching and flexibility routines can improve joint range of motion, reducing the risk of muscle strains or other injuries during workouts.

- Recovery: Flexibility exercises, like yoga or stretching, aid in post-workout recovery. They help reduce muscle soreness and promote relaxation.

- Balance and Posture: Improved flexibility can enhance balance and posture, which are vital for overall well-being.

The significance of exercise in maintaining and increasing muscle mass is substantial. Resistance training is the primary driver of muscle growth, directly stimulating muscle fibers to increase in size and strength. Cardiovascular exercise and flexibility routines play complementary roles in overall fitness. Cardiovascular exercise supports heart health, burns calories, and enhances endurance, while flexibility routines aid in injury prevention and recovery. A well-rounded fitness program that includes all these elements is essential for preserving and increasing muscle mass and overall health.

How can individuals determine their optimal caloric intake and macro-nutrient ratios?

Determining your optimal caloric intake and macro-nutrient ratios is essential for achieving your fitness and nutritional goals. These values are highly individual and depend on factors such as age, gender, activity level, and specific objectives, whether it's weight loss, muscle gain, or maintenance. Here's a detailed explanation of how individuals can calculate their daily calorie needs and find the ideal balance of carbohydrates, proteins, and fats:

1. Calculate Daily Caloric Needs:

a. Basal Metabolic Rate (BMR): BMR represents the number of calories your body needs at rest to maintain basic functions like breathing, circulation, and cell production. Several equations can estimate BMR, with the Harris-Benedict equation being one of the most widely used. The equation differs for men and women:

- For Men: BMR = 88.362 + (13.397 × weight in kg) + (4.799 × height in cm) - (5.677 × age in years)
- For Women: BMR = 447.593 + (9.247 × weight in kg) + (3.098 × height in cm) - (4.330 ×

age in years)

b. Total Daily Energy Expenditure (TDEE): Once you have your BMR, you need to factor in your activity level. The TDEE represents the total calories you burn daily, including your physical activity. Use the following multipliers to estimate your TDEE:

- Sedentary (Little to no exercise): BMR × 1.2
- Lightly active (Light exercise or sports 1-3 days a week): BMR × 1.375
- Moderately active (Moderate exercise or sports 3-5 days a week): BMR × 1.55
- Very active (Hard exercise or sports 6-7 days a week): BMR × 1.725
- Super active (Very hard exercise, physical job, or training twice a day): BMR × 1.9

c. Weight Goals: To determine the number of calories needed for weight loss or gain, you must create a calorie deficit or surplus. Typically, a 500-calorie deficit per day leads to a safe rate of weight loss (about 1 pound per week), while a 500-calorie surplus can support muscle gain. Adjust your daily caloric intake accordingly.

2. Determine Ideal Macro-nutrient Ratios:

a. Proteins: Proteins are essential for muscle repair and growth. A common recommendation is to consume 10-35% of daily calories from protein. A more precise guideline is to aim for around 1.2 to 2.2 grams of protein per kilogram of body weight, depending on your activity level and goals.

b. Carbohydrates: Carbohydrates are the body's primary energy source. They should make up about 45-65% of your daily caloric intake. The proportion can be adjusted based on your activity level, with more carbs needed for high-intensity exercise.

c. Fats: Dietary fats are necessary for overall health. They should contribute around 20-35% of your daily calories. Focus on healthy fats like those found in avocados, nuts, and olive oil.

3. Monitor and Adjust:

a. Tracking: Use a food diary or a mobile app to monitor your food intake. Track your macro-nutrient consumption to ensure you're meeting your goals.

b. Regular Assessment: Periodically reassess your calorie and macro-nutrient intake based on your progress and any changes in your goals or activity levels.

c. Consult a Professional: If you have specific

dietary needs, fitness goals, or underlying health conditions, consider consulting with a registered dietitian or nutritionist. They can provide personalized guidance and help you create a nutrition plan that aligns with your objectives.

Calculating your daily caloric needs and determining your ideal macro-nutrient ratios is a critical step in managing your nutrition for various fitness and health goals. It requires understanding your BMR, estimating your TDEE based on activity level, and tailoring your macro-nutrient ratios to meet your specific objectives. Regular monitoring and adjustments are essential for long-term success in achieving your nutritional goals.

What are the best exercises for muscle building?

The best exercises for muscle building are those that primarily engage your muscle fibers and provide the stimulus for hypertrophy (muscle growth). These exercises are typically part of resistance training, which can involve various techniques and workout programs. The choice of exercises can vary based on your goals, experience level, and equipment available. Here's a detailed explanation of various resistance training techniques, exercises, and workout programs that promote muscle growth:

1. Compound Exercises:

Compound exercises work multiple muscle groups simultaneously, making them highly effective for muscle building. They promote greater muscle activation and hormonal response. Examples include:

- Squats: Target the quadriceps, hamstrings, glutes, and lower back.
- Dead-lifts: Engage the lower back, hamstrings, glutes, and grip strength.
- Bench Press: Works the chest, shoulders, and triceps.
- Pull-Ups/Chin-Ups: Focus on the back, biceps,

and shoulders.
- Rows: Target the upper back, traps, and biceps.

2. Isolation Exercises:

Isolation exercises target specific muscle groups and are effective for fine-tuning and targeting particular areas. Examples include:

- Bicep Curls: Isolate the biceps.
- Tricep Extensions: Target the triceps.
- Leg Curls: Work the hamstrings.
- Leg Extensions: Isolate the quadriceps.

3. Free Weights:

Free weights, such as dumbbells and barbells, require greater stability and activate stabilizing muscles, making them ideal for muscle building. You can perform exercises like: (See Support Products Page.)

- Dumbbell Presses: Dumbbell bench press, overhead press.
- Barbell Rows: Bent-over rows, T-bar rows.
- Dumbbell Lunges: Target the legs.
- Barbell Shrugs: Develop the traps.

4. Bodyweight Exercises:

Bodyweight exercises can be effective for muscle

building, especially for beginners. These include:

- Push-Ups: Target the chest, shoulders, and triceps.
- Dips: Work the triceps and chest.
- Bodyweight Squats: Engage the legs.
- Pull-Ups/Chin-Ups: Focus on the upper body.

5. Machines:

Weight machines can be beneficial, especially for those new to resistance training. They provide stability and allow for controlled movements. Common machine exercises include: (See Support Products Page.)

- Leg Press: Target the lower body.
- Chest Fly Machine: Work the chest muscles.
- Lat Pulldown: Engage the upper back and biceps.

6. Compound Movement Programs:

Several workout programs focus on compound movements and are popular for muscle building:

- 5x5 StrongLifts: Emphasizes five sets of five reps for key compound exercises.
- Push-Pull-Legs (PPL): Splits workouts into push (e.g., chest and triceps), pull (e.g., back and biceps), and legs.

- Full-Body Workouts: Incorporate a variety of compound exercises in each session.

7. Progressive Overload:

The principle of progressive overload is key for muscle growth. To build muscle, gradually increase the weight, reps, or sets of your exercises. This ensures that you consistently challenge your muscles.

8. Rest and Recovery:

Allowing adequate time for rest and recovery is crucial. Overtraining can hinder muscle growth, so ensure you have rest days between intense workouts to let your muscles repair and grow.

9. Nutrition:

Adequate nutrition is essential for muscle growth. Ensure you're consuming enough protein and calories to support muscle repair and growth.

The best exercises for muscle building encompass a variety of resistance training techniques, exercises, and workout programs. The key is to incorporate compound movements, progressive overload, and proper rest and nutrition to optimize your muscle-building efforts. Tailor your program to your specific goals and adapt it as you gain experience and your objectives evolve.

How often should people work out to maintain muscle mass?

The frequency of workouts is a crucial factor in maintaining and building muscle mass. To determine how often you should work out to achieve your muscle-building goals, it's important to understand the concept of workout frequency, the role of recovery periods, and the necessity of incorporating rest days into your routine. Here's a detailed explanation:

1. Workout Frequency:

Workout frequency refers to how often you engage in resistance training or muscle-building exercises. The ideal frequency can vary depending on your goals, experience level, and individual factors. Here are some key considerations:

- **Beginners:** For those new to resistance training, 2-3 workouts per week can be effective for maintaining and building muscle. This allows time for your body to adapt and recover.

- **Intermediate and Advanced:** As you progress, you may benefit from more frequent workouts, typically 3-6 times per week. A split routine, where you target different muscle groups on different days, can be effective.

- Volume and Intensity: Adjusting the volume (number of sets and repetitions) and intensity (weight lifted) of your workouts can help determine the appropriate workout frequency. Heavier weights and higher volume may require more recovery time.

2. Recovery Periods:

Recovery periods between workouts are crucial for muscle repair and growth. During resistance training, you create small tears in muscle fibers. The recovery process involves repairing these tears, which leads to muscle hypertrophy (growth). Here's how recovery periods contribute to muscle maintenance and growth:

- Muscle Repair: Recovery periods allow your body to repair damaged muscle tissue. Adequate time between workouts ensures that this repair process is complete.

- Central Nervous System Recovery: Intense resistance training can fatigue the central nervous system. Providing sufficient recovery time allows your nervous system to recuperate, reducing the risk of overtraining.

- **Prevention of Overtraining:** Overtraining can lead to muscle breakdown and hinder progress. Rest and recovery periods are essential to avoid overtraining and its negative effects on muscle mass.

3. Rest Days:

Rest days are an integral part of any muscle-building routine. They are designated days when you don't engage in intense resistance training. Here's why rest days are essential:

- **Muscle Recovery:** Rest days provide an opportunity for your muscles to recover fully from the stress of resistance training. This promotes muscle repair and growth.

- **Injury Prevention:** Overuse injuries are more likely to occur if you don't incorporate rest days. Rest days help reduce the risk of overuse injuries, such as strains and tendonitis.

- **Mental and Psychological Well-being:** Taking rest days can help prevent burnout and mental fatigue associated with intense workouts. This contributes to a more sustainable, long-term approach to fitness.

4. Personalization:

The ideal workout frequency, recovery periods, and rest days can vary from person to person. Factors such as age, genetics, fitness level, and goals play a role in determining the best approach for you. Listen to your body and adapt your workout routine accordingly.

How often people should work out to maintain muscle mass depends on their individual factors and goals. The right balance involves finding a frequency that allows for adequate recovery and includes rest days to prevent overtraining. Progressive overload and proper nutrition also play key roles in building and maintaining muscle mass. It's essential to consult with a fitness professional or personal trainer if you have specific goals or concerns related to your workout frequency and muscle-building routine.

What are the signs of over-training, and how can they be prevented?

Overtraining, also known as overtraining syndrome (OTS), can have detrimental effects on both physical and mental well-being. It occurs when the intensity and volume of exercise exceed the body's ability to recover. Recognizing the signs of overtraining and taking preventive measures are crucial for maintaining a healthy and sustainable fitness routine. Here's a detailed explanation of the signs of overtraining and strategies for prevention:

Signs of Overtraining:

1. Decreased Performance: One of the earliest signs is a noticeable decline in exercise performance. You may struggle to lift weights or perform at previous levels of intensity.

2. Chronic Fatigue: Overtraining often leads to chronic fatigue that doesn't improve with rest. You may feel tired all the time and have difficulty recovering between workouts.

3. Insomnia: Sleep disturbances, such as difficulty falling asleep or staying asleep, are common signs of overtraining. Quality sleep is essential for recovery.

4. Mood Changes: Overtraining can result in mood swings, irritability, and increased stress. Hormonal imbalances may contribute to these mood changes.

5. Persistent Soreness: Experiencing persistent muscle soreness or joint pain, unrelated to specific injuries, is a sign of overtraining. The body doesn't have enough time to repair and recover.

6. Weakened Immune System: Frequent illnesses, like colds and infections, can be indicative of a weakened immune system caused by overtraining.

7. Decreased Appetite: Overtraining can suppress appetite, leading to inadequate nutritional intake, which further impairs recovery.

8. Changes in Heart Rate: A consistently elevated resting heart rate or changes in heart rate variability may be a sign of overtraining.

9. Decreased Motivation: A loss of interest or motivation in exercise can be a result of overtraining and the mental stress it can cause.

Preventing Overtraining:

1. Balanced Training: Create a well-structured workout plan that balances intensity, volume, and frequency. Incorporate rest days and recovery weeks into your routine to allow for physical and mental recuperation.

2. Progressive Overload: Gradually increase the intensity and volume of your workouts. Avoid sudden, drastic changes in your training plan.

3. Nutrition: Ensure you're consuming enough calories, especially when increasing physical activity. Proper nutrition supports muscle recovery and overall well-being.

4. Rest and Recovery: Prioritize rest and recovery. Include active recovery days, where you engage in low-intensity activities like walking or yoga.

5. Quality Sleep: Aim for 7-9 hours of quality sleep each night. A good night's sleep is essential for recovery.

6. Listen to Your Body: Pay attention to the signals your body is sending. If you experience signs of overtraining, don't ignore them. Adjust your training and recovery accordingly.

7. Stress Management: Manage stress through techniques like meditation, deep breathing, and relaxation exercises. Stress can exacerbate the effects of overtraining.

8. Variation: Incorporate variety into your workouts to prevent monotony and reduce the risk of overtraining. Include different exercises, training modalities, and sports.

9. Professional Guidance: If you suspect overtraining or have specific concerns, consider consulting with a fitness professional or a healthcare provider. They can help you assess your training plan and make necessary adjustments.

Overtraining is a real concern for anyone engaged in regular exercise. Recognizing the signs of overtraining and taking preventive measures is essential for maintaining a sustainable fitness routine and preventing the negative effects it can have on physical and mental health. A balanced approach to exercise, proper nutrition, rest, and stress management are key components of avoiding overtraining.

How does the body recover from workouts?

Recovery is a crucial aspect of any workout routine, as it's during the recovery phase that your body repairs and adapts to the stress placed on it during exercise. Understanding the processes of muscle repair, glycogen replenishment, and the role of sleep in recovery can help you optimize your recovery strategies. Here's a detailed explanation of how the body recovers from workouts:

1. Muscle Repair and Growth:

a. Muscle Microtrauma: When you engage in resistance training or intense physical activity, you create microscopic damage in your muscle fibers. This damage, also known as muscle microtrauma, is a normal response to exercise.

b. Inflammatory Response: The body responds to this microtrauma with an inflammatory process. Inflammatory markers like cytokines are released, which play a role in signaling the repair process.

c. Protein Synthesis: Muscle repair and growth primarily occur through a process called muscle protein synthesis (MPS). MPS is the creation of new muscle proteins, particularly myofibrillar proteins that make up the contractile units of muscle fibers.

d. Amino Acid Utilization: Amino acids, the building blocks of protein, are essential for muscle repair and growth. Dietary protein provides the necessary amino acids, and consuming protein-rich foods post-workout helps initiate MPS by supplying the raw materials needed for muscle protein synthesis.

2. Glycogen Replenishment:

a. Glycogen Depletion: During exercise, especially endurance activities or high-intensity workouts, your body uses stored carbohydrates in the form of glycogen as a primary energy source. As a result, glycogen stores in muscles and the liver are depleted.

b. Carbohydrate Intake: Post-workout, consuming carbohydrates is essential for glycogen replenishment. Carbohydrates are broken down into glucose and stored as glycogen for future use.

c. Timing: The post-workout window is often referred to as the "glycogen window," where your body is more efficient at replenishing glycogen stores. Consuming carbohydrates within this window can accelerate the process.

3. Role of Sleep in Recovery:

a. Muscle Repair: While you sleep, your body focuses on repairing and rebuilding tissues, including muscle. During deep sleep stages, growth hormone levels rise, stimulating muscle repair and growth.

b. Neurological Recovery: Sleep is crucial for neurological recovery. It helps the central nervous system recover from the demands of exercise, reducing the risk of overtraining and injury.

c. Hormone Balance: Sleep plays a vital role in hormone regulation, including those that affect muscle growth and recovery. Insufficient sleep can disrupt hormone balance and hinder recovery.

d. Mental and Emotional Restoration: Sleep is also essential for mental and emotional well-being. It helps reduce stress and improves mood, which indirectly supports physical recovery.

4. Hydration and Nutrition:

Proper hydration and nutrition are essential for recovery. Water is necessary for many physiological processes, including muscle function. Adequate intake of vitamins and minerals supports various metabolic processes related to muscle growth and recovery.

5. Active Recovery:
Light physical activity on rest days can aid recovery by promoting blood flow to muscles and reducing stiffness. Activities like walking, cycling, or yoga are suitable for active recovery.

The body recovers from workouts through processes like muscle repair and growth, glycogen replenishment, and the role of sleep in recovery. Proper nutrition, hydration, and active recovery can further support the recovery process. Understanding these mechanisms can help individuals optimize their post-workout routines and make informed choices to enhance recovery and overall fitness progress.

What is the impact of sleep and rest on muscle recovery and overall health?

The impact of sleep and rest on muscle recovery and overall health is profound. Quality sleep, adequate rest, and effective stress management are crucial components of a successful fitness regimen and essential for optimal muscle recovery and overall well-being. Here's a detailed explanation of their importance:

1. Sleep and Muscle Recovery:

a. Hormone Regulation: Sleep plays a crucial role in regulating hormones that impact muscle recovery. Growth hormone, which stimulates muscle growth and repair, is primarily released during deep sleep stages. Additionally, adequate sleep supports testosterone production, another hormone that influences muscle development.

b. Muscle Repair: During sleep, your body focuses on repairing and rebuilding tissues, including muscle. The muscle protein synthesis (MPS) process is most active during sleep, leading to the repair and growth of muscle fibers damaged during exercise.

c. Neurological Recovery: Sleep is essential for the central nervous system to recover from the demands of exercise. Without proper rest, your nervous system can become fatigued, increasing the risk of overtraining and injuries.

d. Inflammation Reduction: Adequate sleep helps control inflammation in the body, which can be elevated after intense workouts. Reducing inflammation is critical for muscle repair and overall health.

2. Rest and Muscle Recovery:

a. Rest Between Workouts: Rest days or rest intervals between workouts are necessary to allow muscles to recover fully. Overexercising or not providing enough time for rest can lead to overtraining, which may result in muscle breakdown and hinder progress.

b. Prevention of Overuse Injuries: Adequate rest is essential for preventing overuse injuries. Rest allows your muscles, tendons, and joints to recover and reduces the risk of strains, tendonitis, and stress fractures.

c. Psychological Well-being: Rest is also essential for mental and emotional well-being. It helps prevent burnout, maintains motivation, and allows you to enjoy your fitness routine, contributing to a more sustainable approach to health and fitness.

3. Stress Management and Muscle Recovery:

a. Stress Hormones: Chronic stress can elevate stress hormones like cortisol, which can have catabolic (muscle-breakdown) effects. Managing stress through techniques like meditation, deep breathing, and relaxation exercises can help reduce the impact of stress on muscle recovery.

b. Overall Health: Stress management is not only important for muscle recovery but also for overall health. High stress levels can lead to a range of health issues, including cardiovascular problems and mental health conditions. These can interfere with your ability to engage in physical activities and negatively impact your muscle recovery and general well-being.

4. Optimizing Nutrition:

Quality sleep and rest are also linked to better nutrition. When well-rested, you're more likely to make healthier food choices and maintain a balanced diet. Inadequate sleep can lead to poor dietary decisions, affecting your energy levels, muscle recovery, and overall health.

5. Chronic Sleep Deprivation:

Chronic sleep deprivation has been associated with various health problems, including obesity, insulin resistance, and cardiovascular diseases. These conditions can indirectly affect muscle recovery and fitness progress.

The impact of sleep and rest on muscle recovery and overall health cannot be overstated. Quality sleep supports hormonal balance, muscle repair, and neurological recovery. Adequate rest between workouts prevents overtraining and overuse injuries. Effective stress management reduces the catabolic effects of stress hormones and promotes overall health. Combining these elements with proper nutrition and a well-structured fitness routine is key to achieving optimal muscle recovery and maintaining overall well-being.

How can individuals manage and prevent workout-related injuries?

Managing and preventing workout-related injuries is essential for maintaining a consistent fitness routine and overall well-being. Injury prevention involves several strategies, including proper warm-ups, cool-downs, and maintaining correct exercise form. Here's a detailed explanation of how individuals can manage and prevent workout-related injuries:

1. Warm-Up:

- Importance: A proper warm-up is essential as it increases blood flow to muscles, raises core body temperature, and prepares the body for more strenuous exercise. It also enhances joint mobility and flexibility.

- Dynamic Stretching: Dynamic stretching involves controlled, repetitive movements that mimic the motions you'll perform during your workout. This helps improve flexibility and range of motion. Examples include leg swings, arm circles, and hip rotations.

- Cardiovascular Warm-Up: Incorporating 5-10 minutes of light aerobic exercise, like jogging or cycling, raises your heart rate and gets your muscles ready for activity.

2. Cool-Down:

- Importance: The cool-down is essential for gradually reducing heart rate and allowing your body to return to a resting state. It helps remove waste products from muscles and reduce the risk of post-workout muscle cramps.

- Static Stretching: After your workout, static stretching can help improve flexibility and relieve muscle tension. Hold stretches for 15-30 seconds per muscle group. Focus on major muscle groups like the quadriceps, hamstrings, calves, and upper body.

- Deep Breathing: Deep, diaphragmatic breathing during the cool-down can promote relaxation and reduce muscle tension.

3. Proper Exercise Form:

- Form and Technique: Maintaining correct form during exercises is crucial for injury prevention. Proper technique ensures that you target the right muscles and avoid unnecessary strain on joints and ligaments.

- Education: If you're unsure about proper form, consider working with a certified personal trainer or fitness professional. They can provide guidance and ensure you're using correct technique.

4. Gradual Progression:

- Overuse Injuries: Avoid overuse injuries by gradually increasing the intensity and volume of your workouts. Sudden, dramatic changes in your routine can lead to injuries.

- Listen to Your Body: Pay attention to your body and recognize when you need rest or adjustments in your training. Pushing through pain or discomfort can lead to injuries.

5. Strength and Flexibility Training:

- Strength Training: Building strength in all major muscle groups can improve joint stability and reduce the risk of injury. Balanced muscle development is key.

- Flexibility Training: Regular flexibility exercises, like yoga or static stretching, can enhance joint mobility and reduce muscle tightness, decreasing the likelihood of injuries.

6. Cross-Training:

- Variety: Incorporate a variety of exercises and

activities into your routine. Cross-training can prevent overuse injuries and provide a more well-rounded fitness program.

7. Footwear and Equipment:

- Proper Gear: Wear appropriate footwear and workout attire. Proper shoes provide support and cushioning for different types of exercise. (See Support Products Page.)

8. Recovery and Rest:

- Recovery Days: Allow for adequate recovery between intense workouts. Overtraining can increase the risk of injuries. Rest days and active recovery can help.

9. Nutrition and Hydration:

- Balanced Diet: Maintain a balanced diet that supports your workouts and promotes overall health. Proper nutrition ensures your body has the necessary nutrients for recovery and injury prevention.

- Hydration: Staying well-hydrated is essential for muscle and joint function. Dehydration can increase the risk of cramps and injuries.

10. Medical Consultation:

- Pre-existing Conditions: If you have pre-existing medical conditions or are recovering from an injury, consult with a healthcare professional or physical therapist to develop a workout plan that accommodates your specific needs.

Managing and preventing workout-related injuries involves a combination of strategies, including proper warm-ups, cool-downs, maintaining correct exercise form, gradual progression, strength and flexibility training, cross-training, using proper gear, allowing for recovery, and staying well-nourished and hydrated. Being attentive to your body, listening to its signals, and seeking guidance when needed are key components of a safe and injury-free fitness journey.

What are the effects of aging on muscle mass and how can it be mitigated?

Aging has significant effects on muscle mass and strength, a phenomenon often referred to as age-related muscle loss or sarcopenia. While these changes are a natural part of the aging process, they can be mitigated and managed through a combination of exercise and nutrition. Here's a detailed explanation of the effects of aging on muscle mass and strategies to counteract it:

Effects of Aging on Muscle Mass and Strength:

1. Loss of Muscle Mass: As individuals age, there is a gradual decline in muscle mass. From the age of 30 or 40, people can lose about 3-8% of their muscle mass per decade. This loss accelerates after the age of 60.

2. Reduced Muscle Strength: Alongside muscle mass loss, there is a decrease in muscle strength. Muscle strength is crucial for functional independence, and a decline in strength can impact activities of daily living.

3. Impaired Muscle Function: Aging can lead to reduced muscle function, including diminished power, endurance, and coordination. These changes can contribute to mobility issues and an

increased risk of falls.

4. Increased Fat Mass: As muscle mass decreases, fat mass may increase, leading to changes in body composition. This shift can have adverse effects on overall health and well-being.

Strategies to Counteract Age-Related Muscle Loss:

1. Resistance Training:

   - Importance: Resistance training, including weight lifting and bodyweight exercises, is a powerful strategy to counteract muscle loss and improve muscle strength.

   - Progressive Overload: To stimulate muscle growth and strength, incorporate progressive overload into your resistance training routine. Gradually increase the weight, reps, or sets over time.

2. Protein Intake:

   - Protein Importance: Protein is a critical component of muscle repair and growth. Older adults should aim to maintain or increase their protein intake to support muscle health. (See Support Products Page.)

- Adequate Protein: Consume protein-rich foods like lean meats, poultry, fish, eggs, dairy, and plant-based sources such as legumes, tofu, and nuts. Protein supplements may be considered, especially for those with dietary limitations.

3. Balanced Nutrition:

- Macro and Micro Nutrients: Maintain a balanced diet with adequate intake of macro-nutrients (carbohydrates, protein, and fats) and micro-nutrients (vitamins and minerals). These support overall health and muscle function. (See Support Products Page.)

4. Hydration:

- Fluid Balance: Staying well-hydrated is essential for muscle and joint function. Dehydration can lead to muscle cramps and fatigue.

5. Adequate Caloric Intake:

- Energy Balance: Consume enough calories to support daily activities and exercise. Avoid excessive caloric restriction, as it can accelerate muscle loss.

6. Cardiovascular Exercise:

- Aerobic Fitness: Cardiovascular exercise, such as walking, cycling, or swimming, complements resistance training by improving cardiovascular health and overall endurance. It can help with daily activities and maintain mobility.

7. Flexibility and Mobility Work:

- Range of Motion: Incorporate stretching and mobility exercises to maintain joint flexibility. This can reduce the risk of injury and improve functional abilities.

8. Regular Exercise Routine:

- Consistency: Consistency is key. Engage in regular exercise and maintain an active lifestyle to support muscle health and overall well-being.

9. Bone Health:

- Bone Strength: Age-related muscle loss is often associated with bone density reduction. Engaging in weight-bearing exercises and ensuring adequate calcium and vitamin D intake can support both muscle and bone health. (See Support Products Page.)

10. Consultation with Healthcare Professionals:

- Individualized Plans: If you have specific concerns or health conditions, consult with a healthcare professional, physical therapist, or registered dietitian to create an individualized plan that addresses your needs and goals.

While aging brings about natural changes in muscle mass and strength, these changes can be mitigated through a combination of resistance training, proper nutrition, hydration, cardiovascular exercise, flexibility work, and maintaining a healthy lifestyle. Staying active and focusing on muscle health is essential for enhancing the quality of life in later years.

What role do hormones play in muscle growth and maintenance?

Hormones play a fundamental role in muscle growth and maintenance. They are the chemical messengers that regulate various physiological processes, including muscle protein synthesis and tissue repair. Three key hormones, in particular, have a significant influence on muscle development: testosterone, growth hormone, and insulin. Here's a detailed explanation of their roles in muscle growth and maintenance:

1. Testosterone: (See Support Products Page.)

- Anabolic Hormone: Testosterone is a male sex hormone, although it's also present in smaller amounts in females. It's a potent anabolic hormone, meaning it promotes the growth and repair of muscle tissue.

- Protein Synthesis: Testosterone increases muscle protein synthesis, which is the process by which new muscle proteins are built. This results in muscle hypertrophy, or the growth of muscle fibers.

- Strength and Power: Testosterone also enhances muscle strength and power, allowing individuals to lift heavier weights and perform more intense workouts.

- Fat Reduction: Testosterone helps reduce body fat, which can further enhance muscle definition and appearance.

2. Growth Hormone (GH): (See Support Products Page.)

- Stimulates Growth: Growth hormone plays a critical role in stimulating the growth and repair of tissues, including muscle tissue.

- Protein Synthesis: GH enhances muscle protein synthesis, promoting muscle growth and maintenance.

- Recovery: It aids in the recovery of damaged muscle fibers, particularly after strenuous exercise or injury.

- Cell Growth and Division: GH also contributes to cell growth and division, allowing for the development of new muscle cells.

- Anti-Catabolic: Growth hormone has anti-catabolic properties, meaning it helps prevent muscle breakdown and aids in muscle preservation.

3. Insulin:

- Nutrient Transport: Insulin is a hormone primarily known for its role in regulating blood sugar. It helps transport glucose and amino acids into muscle cells, which is crucial for energy production and muscle repair.

- Protein Synthesis: Insulin promotes protein synthesis by facilitating the uptake of amino acids into muscle cells, supporting muscle growth and recovery.

- Anti-Catabolic: Like growth hormone, insulin has anti-catabolic effects, preventing muscle breakdown and contributing to muscle maintenance.

Interaction and Synergy:

These hormones don't work in isolation; they interact and complement each other to influence muscle development. For example, testosterone and growth hormone can work synergistically to promote muscle growth. Insulin, by facilitating the uptake of nutrients into muscle cells, can enhance the effects of both testosterone and growth hormone.

How to Optimize Hormonal Influence for Muscle Growth:

- **Strength Training:** Engage in regular resistance training to stimulate the release of these hormones. Compound exercises, such as squats and deadlifts, are particularly effective.

- **Nutrition:** Consume a diet rich in essential nutrients, including protein, carbohydrates, and fats. Protein is vital for muscle repair and growth, while carbohydrates are important for energy and glycogen replenishment.

- **Rest and Sleep:** Ensure you get enough quality sleep, as this is when many of these hormones are most active. During deep sleep stages, growth hormone is released, supporting muscle repair.

- **Balanced Lifestyle:** Minimize chronic stress and lead a balanced lifestyle. Excessive stress and lack of sleep can negatively affect hormone balance.

- **Medical Consultation:** If you have hormonal imbalances or underlying medical conditions, consult with a healthcare professional for guidance and potential hormone replacement therapy (HRT).

Hormones like testosterone, growth hormone, and insulin play a crucial role in muscle growth and maintenance. To optimize their influence, engage in regular strength training, maintain a balanced diet, ensure proper sleep and stress management, and seek medical guidance if necessary. These hormones are essential components in achieving and maintaining muscle health and overall fitness.

What are the health risks of extreme diets and supplements for muscle growth?

Extreme diets and excessive supplementation in the pursuit of muscle growth can pose significant health risks. While the desire to achieve quick and dramatic results is common, it's important to be aware of the potential dangers associated with extreme approaches. Here's a detailed explanation of the health risks and the importance of a balanced approach to muscle growth:

Health Risks of Extreme Diets and Supplements:

1. Nutritional Deficiencies: Extreme diets that severely restrict food groups or caloric intake can lead to nutrient deficiencies. Inadequate nutrition can negatively impact overall health and impair muscle growth and recovery.

2. Metabolic Issues: Very low-calorie diets can slow down the metabolism, making it harder to maintain or build muscle. Prolonged calorie restriction can also lead to muscle loss.

3. Dehydration: Extreme diets may result in dehydration, which can impair muscle function and hinder performance during workouts. Dehydration can also lead to other health issues.

4. Electrolyte Imbalance: Severely restricting food groups can disrupt the balance of essential electrolytes, such as sodium, potassium, and calcium, which are crucial for muscle and nerve function.

5. Gastrointestinal Problems: Extreme diets can cause gastrointestinal distress, including constipation, diarrhea, and nutrient malabsorption.

6. Muscle Breakdown: Insufficient caloric intake and a lack of protein can lead to muscle breakdown, counteracting the goal of muscle growth.

7. Bone Health: Inadequate nutrition can compromise bone health, increasing the risk of fractures and injuries during exercise.

8. Hormonal Imbalances: Extreme dieting can disrupt hormonal balance, leading to issues such as low testosterone or irregular menstrual cycles. Hormonal imbalances can impede muscle growth and overall well-being.

9. Supplement Overuse: Excessive use of supplements, such as protein powders, creatine, or anabolic steroids, can have serious side effects. Anabolic steroids, for instance, can lead to liver damage, cardiovascular problems, and

psychological issues.

10. Psychological Strain: Extreme dieting and the pursuit of unrealistic body standards can contribute to mental health issues, including eating disorders and body dysmorphia.

The Importance of a Balanced Approach:

1. Nutrient-Dense Diet: A balanced approach to nutrition is essential. Consume a variety of nutrient-dense foods, including lean protein sources, complex carbohydrates, healthy fats, fruits, and vegetables. This approach provides the necessary nutrients for muscle growth and overall health.

2. Moderate Caloric Surplus: To promote muscle growth, aim for a moderate caloric surplus. Consuming slightly more calories than your daily needs can support muscle development without excessive fat gain.

3. Protein Intake: Ensure you're getting enough high-quality protein to support muscle repair and growth. Protein supplements may be useful for convenience but should not replace whole foods. (See Support Products Page.)

4. Hydration: Stay well-hydrated to support muscle function, recovery, and overall health.

5. Gradual Progression: Avoid rapid and extreme changes in your exercise and diet routines. Gradual progression is more sustainable and less likely to lead to imbalances and injuries.

6. Rest and Recovery: Prioritize rest and recovery. Overtraining can lead to muscle breakdown and injuries. Rest days and sufficient sleep are essential.

7. Professional Guidance: If you're uncertain about your dietary and exercise plan, consult with a registered dietitian, personal trainer, or healthcare provider. They can help you create a balanced and effective approach tailored to your goals.

Extreme diets and excessive supplementation for muscle growth come with serious health risks. A balanced approach to nutrition, exercise, and lifestyle is the safest and most effective way to achieve and maintain muscle health. It's essential to prioritize long-term well-being over short-term, unsustainable methods.

How can individuals set and track fitness goals?

Setting and tracking fitness goals is essential for progress, motivation, and achieving desired results in your fitness journey. It provides a clear direction and helps you stay accountable. Here's a detailed explanation of how individuals can set and track fitness goals effectively:

Setting Fitness Goals:

1. Define Clear and Specific Goals:

   - Your goals should be specific and well-defined. Rather than a vague goal like "get fit," specify what you want to achieve, such as "lose 10 pounds," "run a 5k in under 30 minutes," or "increase bench press strength by 20%."

2. Set Realistic and Achievable Goals:

   - Your goals should be attainable based on your current fitness level and lifestyle. Unrealistic goals can lead to frustration and demotivation.

3. Establish Short-Term and Long-Term Goals:

   - Short-term goals provide stepping stones to your long-term objectives. Breaking down larger goals into smaller, achievable milestones makes progress more manageable.

4. Prioritize Health and Function:

   - While aesthetics and weight loss are common goals, don't neglect health and functional goals, such as improving cardiovascular fitness, flexibility, or balance.

5. Consider Your Interests:

   - Choose activities and goals that align with your interests. Enjoying your fitness routine makes it more likely that you'll stick with it.

6. Write Down Your Goals:

   - Putting your goals in writing makes them more tangible and can improve commitment and accountability.

Tracking Fitness Goals:

1. Keep a Workout Journal: (See Support Products Page.)

   - Record your workouts, including exercises, sets, reps, and weights lifted. This allows you to track your progress and identify areas for improvement.

2. Use Fitness Apps and Wearables:

   - Many apps and wearable devices track your workouts, steps, and other fitness metrics. They provide data on your activity levels and can help you monitor your progress.

3. Measure Body Composition:

   - Tracking body composition metrics, such as weight, body fat percentage, and muscle mass, can provide valuable insights into your progress. Keep in mind that progress isn't solely about the number on the scale; changes in body composition are often more meaningful.

4. Assess Performance Improvements:

   - Regularly evaluate performance metrics related to your specific fitness goals. This could include time for a 5k run, the amount of weight lifted, or the number of push-ups completed.

5. Revisit and Adjust Goals:

   - Periodically review your goals and adjust them as needed. If you've achieved a goal, set a new one to continue progressing.

6. Seek Professional Guidance:

- Consider consulting with a fitness trainer, nutritionist, or other experts for objective assessments and guidance. They can provide valuable feedback and help you refine your goals.

7. Celebrate Milestones:

- Recognize and celebrate your achievements, both big and small. Positive reinforcement can boost motivation.

8. Stay Consistent:

- Consistency is key. Staying on track with your fitness routine and tracking your progress regularly will help you achieve your goals.

9. Stay Accountable:

- Share your goals with a friend, workout partner, or an online fitness community to create a sense of accountability and support.

10. Stay Flexible:

- While setting goals is important, be flexible in your approach. Life can be unpredictable, and sometimes you may need to adjust your goals to accommodate changes in circumstances.

Setting and tracking fitness goals is a crucial part of any fitness journey. Clear and specific goals, combined with effective tracking methods, can help you stay motivated, make progress, and achieve your desired results. Remember that goals should be realistic, flexible, and aligned with your interests and overall well-being.

What are the psychological aspects of maintaining muscle mass and fitness?

The psychological aspects of maintaining muscle mass and fitness are often underestimated but are crucial for both short-term and long-term success. Addressing these aspects, including motivation, discipline, and mental well-being, is essential for achieving and sustaining fitness goals. Here's a detailed explanation of each of these psychological factors:

1. Motivation:

- Intrinsic vs. Extrinsic: Motivation can be intrinsic (driven by internal factors, like a genuine love for exercise) or extrinsic (external factors, like the desire to impress others). Intrinsic motivation tends to be more sustainable and beneficial for long-term fitness.

- Setting Clear Goals: Clearly defined fitness goals provide motivation. Whether it's losing weight, running a marathon, or gaining muscle, having specific objectives to work toward keeps you motivated.

- Progress Tracking: Monitoring your progress and celebrating small achievements along the way can boost motivation. Use fitness apps, journals, or social support to help with tracking.

- Visualization: Visualize your fitness goals and imagine how you'll feel when you achieve them. Visualization can reinforce motivation and make your goals seem more attainable.

- Accountability: Sharing your goals with a workout partner, trainer, or a supportive community can help maintain motivation. The social aspect and sense of accountability can be powerful motivators.

2. Discipline:

- Consistency: Discipline is the ability to stick to your fitness routine even when you don't feel motivated. Regular workouts, proper nutrition, and adequate rest require discipline.

- Establishing Habits: Turning fitness into a habit can reduce the reliance on motivation. Over time, it becomes a part of your daily life, making it easier to maintain muscle mass and fitness.

- Resisting Temptations: Discipline involves resisting temptations that might derail your progress, such as unhealthy foods or skipping workouts.

- Overcoming Plateaus: Plateaus are a normal part

of any fitness journey. Discipline is what pushes you through these periods, making you continue your efforts to break through and see progress.

3. Mental Well-being:

- Mind-Body Connection: Mental well-being is closely linked to physical health. Regular exercise has been shown to reduce symptoms of anxiety and depression, improving overall mental health.

- Stress Management: Exercise and fitness activities can act as stress relievers. A well-structured fitness program can help you manage stress and maintain emotional well-being.

- Body Image and Self-esteem: Maintaining muscle mass and fitness can boost self-esteem and promote a positive body image. It's essential to focus on overall health and well-being rather than just appearance.

- Mental Toughness: Building mental toughness is vital for maintaining fitness. It's about developing resilience and the ability to push through physical and mental challenges.

- Balancing Rest and Recovery: Mental well-being also involves understanding the importance of rest and recovery. Overtraining can lead to burnout and negatively affect your mental state.

- Positive Self-talk: Practice positive self-talk and avoid negative self-criticism. Encourage yourself and focus on your achievements, no matter how small they may seem.

- Mindfulness and Relaxation: Incorporating mindfulness techniques and relaxation practices, such as meditation, can improve mental well-being and help manage stress.

The psychological aspects of maintaining muscle mass and fitness are critical for achieving and sustaining your goals. Motivation, discipline, and mental well-being all play integral roles. Developing these psychological factors alongside your physical training can lead to a more successful and fulfilling fitness journey. Remember that it's essential to view fitness as a holistic endeavor that benefits both your physical and mental health.

The Spectrum of Organ Regeneration in the Human Body

The regenerative capacity of organs in the human body varies significantly. Some organs can regenerate or repair themselves relatively quickly, while others have limited regenerative abilities or cannot regenerate at all. Here's a general overview of the regenerative capacities of some key organs:

1. Skin: The skin is the body's largest organ and has a high regenerative capacity. It constantly renews itself, and minor injuries, like cuts and scrapes, can heal within days to weeks.

2. Liver: The liver is known for its remarkable regenerative abilities. It can regenerate and return to its normal size and function within a matter of months after injury or partial removal.

3. Bone: Bone tissue has a good regenerative capacity. Fractured bones typically heal in a matter of weeks to a few months, depending on the severity of the injury.

4. Blood: Blood cells, including red blood cells, white blood cells, and platelets, are continually being produced by the bone marrow. This ongoing regeneration maintains the blood's functionality.

5. Intestinal Epithelium: The lining of the small intestine, which is composed of rapidly dividing cells, has a high regenerative capacity. It can renew itself every few days.

6. Lungs: The lungs have limited regenerative capacity. While some regeneration can occur, it is not sufficient to fully repair major damage caused by conditions like emphysema or extensive scarring.

7. Heart: The heart has limited regenerative capacity. While it can replace some damaged tissue with scar tissue, it cannot fully regenerate lost or damaged cardiac muscle cells. However, there is ongoing research into stimulating heart regeneration.

8. Nervous System: The central nervous system, including the brain and spinal cord, has very limited regenerative capacity. Once neurons are damaged or lost, they typically do not regenerate. However, the peripheral nervous system (nerves outside the central nervous system) can regenerate to some extent.

9. Kidneys: The kidneys have some ability to repair minor damage, but their regenerative capacity is limited. Severe damage to kidney tissue can lead to permanent loss of function.

It's important to note that the regenerative capacity of these organs can be influenced by various factors, such as age, overall health, and the extent of damage or injury. Some ongoing medical research aims to enhance regenerative capabilities in certain organs and tissues, but for now, the regenerative capacity of many organs remains limited.

Muscle Regeneration and Recovery

Factors, Timelines, and the DOMS Experience

The regeneration of human muscles after exercise or injury can vary depending on several factors, including the type and extent of muscle damage, an individual's age, overall health, nutrition, and the specific muscle groups involved. Generally, it can take several days to several weeks for muscles to regenerate and repair themselves. Here are some guidelines:

1. Microscopic Muscle Damage

Eccentric Exercise

When you engage in strenuous exercise or activities that cause microscopic muscle damage, such as intense weightlifting or eccentric exercises (lengthening contractions), it may take around 24 to 48 hours for the initial repair and recovery process to begin. This process involves inflammation and the activation of satellite cells to repair and strengthen the damaged muscle fibers.

Let's delve into more detail about the concept of microscopic muscle damage and the initial repair and recovery process, especially in the context of eccentric exercise.

a. Microscopic Muscle Damage:

- Microscopic muscle damage refers to the small-scale structural changes that occur within muscle fibers when they are subjected to intense or strenuous exercise, particularly eccentric exercises. Eccentric exercises involve lengthening contractions of the muscle, such as the lowering phase of a bicep curl, descending a flight of stairs, or performing negative repetitions in weightlifting.

- During eccentric exercise, the muscle is actively lengthening while still under tension. This places significant mechanical stress on the muscle fibers.

b. Initial Response to Exercise:

- After engaging in strenuous or eccentric exercise, the muscle fibers experience mechanical stress and microscopic damage. This damage can manifest as the disruption of muscle cell membranes and the breakdown of contractile proteins within the muscle fibers.

- Almost immediately after exercise, the

body initiates an acute inflammatory response as part of the initial repair and recovery process. This inflammation is a natural and necessary reaction to the damage sustained by the muscle tissue.

- The inflammatory response serves multiple purposes:

- It helps clear away cellular debris and damaged tissue.

- It brings immune cells to the site of damage to initiate repair.

- It activates satellite cells, which are a type of muscle stem cell located in the muscle tissue.

c. Satellite Cells and Repair:

- Satellite cells are vital players in the process of muscle repair and regeneration. When muscle fibers are damaged, these satellite cells become activated.

- Activated satellite cells:

- Multiply and proliferate, creating a pool of new muscle cell precursors.

- Fuse with existing muscle fibers, helping to repair and regenerate the damaged muscle tissue.

- Promote the synthesis of new muscle proteins to strengthen the muscle fibers.

d. Inflammation and Recovery:

- In the hours and days following strenuous exercise, the inflammatory response gradually subsides as the repair process continues.

- The initial inflammation, while it may cause temporary discomfort or soreness, is a crucial part of the recovery process.

- As the muscle tissue repairs, it may become stronger and more resilient than before to better handle future bouts of similar exercise.

e. Timing of Recovery:

- The initial stages of muscle repair and recovery, including the activation of satellite cells and the inflammatory response, can take around 24 to 48 hours to initiate after strenuous exercise. This is why it's common to experience muscle soreness, known as delayed onset muscle soreness (DOMS), a day or two after intense workouts.

- It's important to note that the timeline for full recovery and adaptation of muscle tissue spans a more extended period of weeks and months of consistent training, as discussed in the previous response.

When you engage in strenuous exercise, especially eccentric exercise that causes microscopic muscle damage, the body's initial response involves inflammation and the activation of satellite cells. These processes are essential for the repair and strengthening of damaged muscle fibers. While the immediate repair process begins within 24 to 48 hours, the full adaptation and growth of muscles occur over a more extended period with consistent training and recovery.

2. Soreness and Inflammation:

After intense exercise, you may experience muscle soreness and inflammation, often referred to as delayed onset muscle soreness (DOMS). DOMS typically peaks within 24 to 72 hours after exercise and may gradually subside over the next few days.

Let's explore delayed onset muscle soreness (DOMS) in more detail:

a. What is DOMS?

- DOMS stands for "Delayed Onset Muscle Soreness." It is a common and temporary condition characterized by muscle pain and discomfort that occurs after strenuous or unfamiliar physical activity, especially when you engage in exercises that your muscles are not accustomed to.

- DOMS is often associated with eccentric exercise, where the muscles lengthen under tension, such as during the lowering phase of weightlifting exercises or during activities that involve a lot of downhill or downhill running.

- It is important to note that DOMS is distinct from acute muscle soreness, which is the immediate discomfort or burning sensation you may feel during or right after intense exercise.

b. Symptoms of DOMS:

- DOMS typically manifests as muscle pain, stiffness, and tenderness in the affected muscle groups.

- You may experience reduced range of motion in the joints associated with the sore muscles.

- Swelling and minor inflammation in the affected area can also occur.

c. Timeline of DOMS:

- DOMS does not typically develop immediately after exercise but instead has a delayed onset. It usually peaks within 24 to 72 hours following the exercise session.

- The intensity of DOMS can vary depending on several factors, including the type and intensity of the exercise, an individual's fitness level, and how well they recover and manage post-exercise soreness.

d. Causes of DOMS:

- The exact mechanisms behind DOMS are not fully understood, but it is believed to be related to the microscopic damage and inflammation that occurs within muscle fibers as a result of intense exercise.

- Factors that may contribute to the development of DOMS include:

- Eccentric muscle contractions: Exercises that involve lengthening muscle contractions, such as lowering a weight slowly, are more likely to cause DOMS.

- Mechanical stress: The mechanical stress experienced by muscle fibers during eccentric contractions can lead to structural damage and inflammation.

- Muscle imbalances: If certain muscle groups are weaker than others, they may be more susceptible to DOMS during exercises that target those specific muscles.

- Muscle fatigue: Overexertion, inadequate warm-up, or performing a high volume of exercise can contribute to the development of DOMS.

e. Management of DOMS:

- DOMS is usually a self-limiting condition, meaning it will improve on its own as the body completes the repair and recovery process.

- While there is no guaranteed way to prevent DOMS, there are strategies that can help alleviate symptoms and promote recovery, including:

- Gentle stretching and low-intensity exercise to increase blood flow to the sore muscles.

- Rest and allowing time for the muscles to recover.

- Applying ice or heat to the affected area.

- Over-the-counter pain relievers, if recommended by a healthcare professional.

- Maintaining proper hydration and nutrition to support muscle recovery.

Delayed onset muscle soreness (DOMS) is a temporary condition characterized by muscle pain and discomfort that occurs after intense or unfamiliar exercise, typically peaking within 24 to 72 hours after the exercise session. It is thought to result from microscopic muscle damage and inflammation. While there is no surefire way to prevent DOMS, it can be managed with rest, gentle movement, and other supportive measures to help ease symptoms and promote recovery.

3. Muscle Protein Synthesis:

The actual regeneration of muscle tissue occurs over several days to weeks. Protein synthesis and muscle repair are ongoing processes. It may take several days for significant regeneration to occur, and the time frame can vary depending on the individual and the extent of muscle damage.

Let's explore the process of muscle protein synthesis (MPS) and its crucial function in the regeneration and repair of muscle tissue.

a. What is Muscle Protein Synthesis (MPS)?

   - Muscle protein synthesis is the process by which the body builds new muscle proteins or repairs existing ones. It is a fundamental aspect of muscle regeneration and adaptation in response to exercise, injury, or other factors.

b. Role of MPS in Muscle Regeneration:

- MPS plays a central role in repairing and rebuilding muscle tissue after it has been damaged, as it provides the necessary raw materials for muscle growth and repair.

- After strenuous exercise or when muscle fibers are damaged, there is an increased demand for protein synthesis to replace or reinforce the damaged muscle proteins.

c. Key Points about Muscle Protein Synthesis:

- Muscle protein synthesis is an ongoing process, and it is especially active during the recovery phase following exercise.

- It involves the incorporation of amino acids into muscle proteins, which are the building blocks of muscle tissue.

- The primary amino acids involved in MPS are essential amino acids, which the body cannot produce on its own and must be obtained through diet or supplementation.

Amino acids are the fundamental building blocks of proteins, including muscle proteins. There are 20 different amino acids that make up proteins, and they can be divided into two main categories: essential amino acids and non-essential amino acids.

Essential Amino Acids (EAAs): These are amino acids that the body cannot produce on its own, so they must be obtained through your diet or supplementation. Essential amino acids play a crucial role in muscle protein synthesis and muscle recovery. The nine essential amino acids are: (See Support Products Page.)

1. Leucine
2. Isoleucine
3. Valine
4. Threonine
5. Methionine
6. Phenylalanine
7. Tryptophan
8. Histidine
9. Lysine

Non-Essential Amino Acids: These amino acids can be synthesized by the body, so they are not considered essential in the diet. However, they also contribute to various physiological processes and protein synthesis. Non-essential amino acids include:

1. Alanine

2. Arginine

3. Asparagine

4. Aspartic acid

5. Cysteine

6. Glutamine

7. Glutamic acid

8. Glycine

9. Proline

10. Serine

11. Tyrosine

In the context of muscle recovery and muscle protein synthesis, it's the essential amino acids, particularly leucine, that are of great importance. Leucine, in particular, plays a central role in initiating the muscle protein synthesis process. It acts as a signal to activate protein synthesis and helps stimulate the growth of muscle tissue.

Supplementing with essential amino acids or branched-chain amino acids (BCAAs), which include leucine, is a common practice among athletes and individuals looking to support muscle recovery and growth. BCAA supplements typically contain three essential amino acids: leucine, isoleucine, and valine. They are often consumed before, during, or after workouts to help provide the necessary building blocks for muscle protein synthesis. (See Support Products Page.)

Regarding specific brands and dosages, it's important to note that the optimal dosage of amino acid supplements can vary based on individual factors, such as body weight, training intensity, and goals. It's recommended to follow the manufacturer's guidelines on the product label for proper dosages. As for specific brands, it's a good idea to choose reputable and well-established brands that adhere to quality standards and provide transparent information about the ingredients in their products.

Remember that while amino acid supplementation can be beneficial, it should not replace a balanced and varied diet that includes a wide range of protein sources, including lean meats, dairy, eggs, legumes, and other whole foods. Additionally, consulting with a healthcare professional or nutritionist can help you determine your specific dietary and supplementation needs based on your fitness goals and individual circumstances.

4. Time Frame of MPS:

   - The time frame for muscle protein synthesis can vary depending on several factors:

- Extent of muscle damage: The more significant the muscle damage, the greater the demand for protein synthesis, which can extend the duration of the process.

- Individual factors: Each person's rate of protein synthesis can be influenced by genetics, age, hormonal factors, and overall health.

- Nutrition and recovery: Consuming adequate protein and calories, as well as getting sufficient rest, can support and optimize the process of MPS.

- Training experience: Individuals who are new to resistance training may experience more rapid gains in muscle protein synthesis compared to experienced athletes.

5. Optimizing Muscle Protein Synthesis:

- To optimize muscle protein synthesis for muscle regeneration and growth, consider the following:

- Protein intake: Ensure you are consuming enough high-quality protein to provide the necessary amino acids for muscle repair and growth. Protein-rich foods like lean meats, dairy, eggs, and plant-based sources can be beneficial. (See Support Products Page.)

- Timing: Consuming protein and essential amino acids around the time of exercise or during the post-exercise recovery window can be particularly advantageous.

- Progressive resistance training: Engage in regular resistance training to stimulate muscle protein synthesis and promote muscle growth.

- Rest and recovery: Allow your muscles to recover through proper sleep, rest days between intense workouts, and stress management.

Optimal nutrition is essential for supporting muscle protein synthesis (MPS). Whole foods that are rich in high-quality protein, along with the right balance of other nutrients, can promote the repair and growth of muscle tissue. Here are some foods that are best for MPS:

1. Lean Meats: Lean cuts of meat like chicken, turkey, and beef are excellent sources of complete protein, which provides all essential amino acids required for MPS.

2. Fish: Fish, such as salmon, tuna, and cod, is not only a great source of protein but also provides healthy omega-3 fatty acids, which can reduce muscle soreness and inflammation.

3. Eggs: Eggs are a complete source of protein, and the protein in eggs is highly bioavailable, making it an excellent choice for supporting MPS.

4. Dairy: Dairy products like Greek yogurt, cottage cheese, and milk are rich in casein and whey protein. Whey protein, in particular, is quickly absorbed and can enhance MPS.

5. Plant-Based Sources: For those who follow a vegetarian or vegan diet, sources of plant-based protein like tofu, tempeh, legumes (beans, lentils, chickpeas), and quinoa can be beneficial. Combining various plant-based protein sources can provide a well-rounded amino acid profile.

6. Nuts and Seeds: Almonds, peanuts, and seeds like chia seeds and flaxseeds contain protein and healthy fats that support muscle recovery.

7. Whole Grains: Whole grains like brown rice, quinoa, and oats can contribute to your protein intake and provide essential nutrients for muscle recovery.

8. Protein Supplements: In addition to whole foods, protein supplements can be a convenient way to ensure you're getting enough protein to support MPS. These supplements can include:

- **Whey Protein:** Whey protein is a rapidly absorbed protein that is particularly effective for post-workout recovery.

- **Casein Protein:** Casein is a slow-digesting protein that can provide a steady supply of amino acids over an extended period, making it a good option before bedtime.

- **Plant-Based Protein:** There are various plant-based protein powders made from sources like peas, rice, hemp, and soy for those who prefer plant-based options.

- **Amino Acid Supplements:** As mentioned earlier, essential amino acids or BCAAs can be used to support MPS, particularly around exercise sessions.

9. Nutrient Timing: Consuming protein-rich foods or supplements in the post-exercise period can be particularly beneficial for MPS. The immediate post-workout window is often referred to as the "anabolic window," during which muscle cells are more receptive to nutrients.

A well-balanced diet that includes a variety of protein sources, along with adequate calories and nutrients, is essential for supporting muscle protein synthesis. Protein-rich foods, as well as protein supplements, can be beneficial for individuals aiming to optimize their muscle recovery and growth. The choice of protein sources and supplements should be based on dietary preferences, nutritional needs, and fitness goals. (See Support Products Page.)

A muscle protein synthesis is the process by which the body builds new muscle proteins and repairs existing ones. It is essential for muscle regeneration and adaptation, especially following strenuous exercise. The time frame for significant muscle regeneration can vary depending on factors such as the extent of muscle damage, individual factors, nutrition, and training experience. By optimizing these factors, individuals can support and enhance the process of muscle protein synthesis to promote muscle growth and recovery.

Recovery and Adaptation

Muscle recovery and adaptation to training can take longer, especially if you're engaged in a regular exercise program to build muscle or improve performance. Over weeks and months of consistent training, your muscles can adapt and grow stronger.

How muscle recovery and adaptation occur over time, especially in the context of a regular exercise program aimed at building muscle and improving performance.

Initial Response to Exercise

- When you engage in resistance training or other forms of strenuous exercise, your muscles experience microtrauma and damage at the cellular level. This is a normal response to the stress placed on the muscles during exercise.

- In response to this stress, there is an acute inflammatory process that begins almost immediately after exercise. This inflammation helps to initiate the repair and regeneration of damaged muscle tissue.

Protein Synthesis and Repair

- In the hours and days following exercise, the body's focus shifts to repairing and rebuilding the damaged muscle fibers. This involves a process called protein synthesis, where new muscle proteins are produced to replace or reinforce the damaged ones.

   - Satellite cells, which are a type of muscle stem cell, play a crucial role in muscle repair. They become activated and help repair and regenerate damaged muscle fibers.

Satellite cells are activated in response to muscle damage or injury, and they play a critical role in muscle repair and regeneration. The activation of satellite cells is a complex process involving various signaling pathways. Here's a simplified explanation of how satellite cells become activated:

1. **Muscle Damage:** Satellite cell activation is triggered by mechanical stress, muscle damage, or inflammation, which can occur as a result of strenuous exercise, eccentric contractions, or other factors that cause damage to muscle fibers.

2. **Release of Growth Factors:** The process of muscle damage leads to the release of growth factors and other signaling molecules in the damaged muscle tissue. These growth factors can

include insulin-like growth factor (IGF-1), hepatocyte growth factor (HGF), and fibroblast growth factor (FGF), among others.

3. **Chemotactic Signals:** The damaged muscle tissue releases chemotactic signals or chemical signals that attract satellite cells to the site of injury. These signals include chemokines and cytokines.

4. **Satellite Cell Activation:** In response to these signals, quiescent satellite cells, which are normally in a dormant state, become activated. Activation involves satellite cells moving from the periphery of muscle fibers to the site of muscle damage.

5. **Proliferation and Differentiation:** Once activated, satellite cells undergo several stages of proliferation and differentiation. They start to multiply, forming a pool of myogenic precursor cells. Some of these cells fuse with existing muscle fibers, contributing to repair and regeneration. Others become myoblasts, which are muscle cell precursors that further differentiate into mature muscle cells.

6. **Muscle Fiber Repair:** The myoblasts and satellite cells that fuse with damaged muscle fibers aid in repairing and reinforcing the muscle tissue. They contribute to the synthesis of new muscle proteins, helping to restore and strengthen the damaged fibers.

7. **Resolution of Inflammation:** As the repair process continues and new muscle fibers are formed, the inflammation in the damaged area gradually subsides. This is part of the body's natural response to the healing process.

It's important to note that the activation of satellite cells is just one aspect of the muscle repair and regeneration process. Proper nutrition, including adequate protein intake, is crucial for providing the building blocks necessary for muscle recovery. Rest, as well as the management of inflammation and muscle soreness, also play significant roles in the overall recovery process after strenuous exercise or muscle injury.

Satellite cells are activated in response to muscle damage, leading to a cascade of events that ultimately results in the repair and regeneration of damaged muscle fibers. This process is tightly regulated and involves the interaction of various signaling molecules and cell types.

Adaptation and Growth

While the initial repair of muscle tissue happens relatively quickly, the adaptation and growth of muscles occur over a more extended period of time.

When you consistently engage in resistance training or regular exercise over weeks and months, your muscles adapt to the increased demands being placed on them. This adaptation can take various forms, such as increased muscle fiber size (hypertrophy) and increased muscle strength.

Key factors contributing to muscle adaptation and growth include

- **Progressive Overload:** To stimulate muscle growth and adaptation, you need to gradually increase the resistance or intensity of your workouts. This progressive overload challenges your muscles to work harder over time.

- **Proper Nutrition:** Adequate nutrition is essential for muscle recovery and growth. Consuming enough protein and calories to support muscle repair and adaptation is crucial.

- **Rest and Recovery:** Sufficient rest and sleep are important for the muscles to recover and adapt. During rest periods, the body continues to repair and strengthen muscle tissue.

- **Individual Variability:** The rate of adaptation and muscle growth varies among individuals. Genetics, age, training history, and other factors can influence how quickly one person sees muscle gains compared to another.

Ongoing Process:

- The process of muscle recovery, adaptation, and growth is ongoing as long as you continue to engage in regular, progressive resistance training or exercise.

- It's important to maintain a consistent workout regimen and make adjustments as needed to continue challenging your muscles and promoting growth.

- It's also worth noting that muscle adaptation and growth may eventually plateau, and further progress may require more advanced training strategies or modifications to your exercise routine.

Muscle recovery and adaptation are complex

processes that occur in response to exercise. The initial repair of damaged muscle tissue happens relatively quickly, but the long-term growth and adaptation of muscles occur over weeks and months of consistent training, provided that you apply the principles of progressive overload, proper nutrition, and adequate rest.

Listening to your body and providing adequate rest between intense workouts is important to allow muscles to recover and regenerate. Overtraining or not allowing enough time for regeneration can lead to injuries or hinder progress. Professional athletes and bodybuilders often follow specific training and recovery routines to optimize muscle regeneration and growth.

Essential Items Needed for Home Exercise

Creating an effective and safe home exercise environment involves having the right equipment and space to support your fitness goals. Here are some essential items needed for home exercise:

1. **Exercise Mat**: A quality exercise mat provides cushioning and support for floor exercises, stretching, and yoga.

2. **Dumbbells or Resistance Bands:** Dumbbells or resistance bands are versatile tools for strength training and can be used to target various muscle groups.

3. **Exercise Ball:** An exercise ball can be used for core strengthening, balance, and flexibility exercises.

4. **Kettlebells:** Kettlebells are excellent for functional strength training and can add variety to your workouts.

5. **Jump Rope:** Jumping rope is a great cardiovascular exercise that doesn't require much space.

6. **Pull-Up Bar:** If you have a doorway with a sturdy frame, a pull-up bar can be used for upper body and core workouts.

7. **Yoga Blocks and Straps:** These props can aid

in yoga practice and flexibility training.

8. **Resistance Tubes or Bands:** These are useful for lower-impact resistance training and can be easily stored.

9. **Stability or Bosu Ball:** These can enhance balance and stability training.

10. **Foam Roller:** Foam rollers are great for self-myofascial release and muscle recovery.

11. **Weight Bench:** A weight bench is essential for more advanced strength training exercises.

12. **Barbell and Weight Plates:** If you have the space and the goal to lift heavier weights, a barbell and weight plates are valuable additions.

13. **Medicine Balls:** Medicine balls can be used for a variety of strength and coordination exercises.

14. **Adjustable Workout Bench:** An adjustable bench can be used for a range of exercises, including incline and decline movements.

15. **Aerobic Step or Platform:** Useful for step aerobics and other cardiovascular workouts.

16. **Full-Length Mirror:** Having a mirror in your workout space can help you monitor your form during exercises.

17. **Music or Entertainment Setup:** Create a motivating atmosphere with a music system, TV, or tablet for workout videos.

18. **Workout Clothing and Shoes:** Comfortable

workout attire and appropriate footwear are essential for safety and comfort.

19. **Timer or Stopwatch:** Useful for interval training and timing rest periods.

20. **Water Bottle:** Staying hydrated during your workouts is crucial.

21. **Fan or Ventilation:** Adequate ventilation can help you stay cool during workouts.

22. **Resistance Bands:** These are convenient for lower-body exercises and stretching.

23. **Gloves and Wrist Wraps:** If you're doing weightlifting, gloves and wrist wraps can protect your hands and wrists.

24. **Fitness Tracker:** A fitness tracker or smartwatch can help you monitor your progress and keep you motivated.

25. **Organizational Storage:** Invest in storage solutions like shelves or bins to keep your equipment organized and easily accessible.

Remember to **choose equipment and items that align with your fitness goals** and the available space in your home. Additionally, make sure to consult with a fitness professional or a trainer if you're new to home workouts to ensure that you're using the equipment correctly and safely.

Support Products

– Use the designated link to be taken to Amazon for product info.

Macro-Nutrients Supplements
https://amzn.to/46Pjr4L
Micro-Nutrients Supplements
https://amzn.to/40dijp2
Branched-Chain Amino Acid (BCAA)
https://amzn.to/3MlIynx
Calcium with Vitamin D
https://amzn.to/46LUibh
Testosterone Booster
https://amzn.to/3Mmuudv
Protein for Muscle Repair
https://amzn.to/46Oyc7Q
Growth Hormone
https://amzn.to/3QyhGTZ
Workout Journal
https://amzn.to/49erdHe
BCAA Amino Acids
https://amzn.to/3QeqcpK
Barbell Weight Set
https://amzn.to/47aKWp8
Home Workout Equipment
https://amzn.to/3Qe9RRR
Workout Shoes
https://amzn.to/45MyMlj
Adjustable Workout Bench
https://amzn.to/49eyTsY

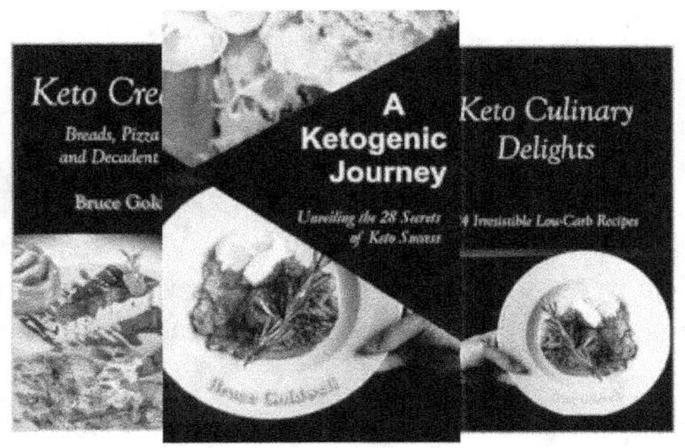

"Keto Culinary Odyssey: Savoring the Low-Carb World"

Step into the flavorful realm of "Keto Culinary Odyssey," a captivating series of books dedicated to the art of the ketogenic lifestyle. These carefully crafted volumes take you on a delicious journey where you'll discover a treasure trove of keto recipes, bread recipes, desserts, and all things related to the low-carb, high-flavor world of Keto.

In each book, you'll unlock the secrets to creating mouthwatering keto dishes that not only satisfy your taste buds but also align with your health and wellness goals. Explore a diverse collection of bread recipes, from hearty loaves to savory rolls, offering the perfect low-carb companions for your culinary adventures.

Indulge in the world of keto desserts that defy expectations, proving that you can enjoy sweet treats while staying in ketosis. From rich and velvety cheesecakes to delectable chocolate creations, these desserts are a testament to the notion that a low-carb lifestyle need not be devoid of

117

culinary delights.

But "Keto Culinary Odyssey" isn't just about recipes. It's a comprehensive exploration of the keto lifestyle, offering guidance, tips, and expert insights to help you thrive in your ketogenic journey. Dive into the science of low-carb living, discover ingredient substitutions, and learn the art of meal planning to make your keto experience seamless and satisfying.

With each book in this series, you'll not only savor the delectable flavors of the keto world but also gain the knowledge and inspiration to make your ketogenic journey a fulfilling and long-lasting adventure. "Keto Culinary Odyssey" invites you to embrace the low-carb lifestyle and unlock the full potential of your culinary creativity while prioritizing your health and well-being.

https://amzn.to/3QegR1k

About The Author

Bruce Goldwell is a self-help/motivational author and creator of two captivating fantasy adventures, "Dragon Keepers" a six book series and "Starfighters Defending Earth" a three book series. He also has books on alternative health, health issues, Keto, weight loss, and the Law of Attraction.

He is an inspiring figure who has overcome significant challenges in his life. As a Vietnam veteran, he experienced homelessness for over ten years. During these difficult times, Bruce developed a compassionate heart and strong desire to uplift others. While living on the streets, he immersed himself in motivational literature at local bookstores, where he found solace in the works of renowned authors such as the creators of Chicken Soup for the Soul, Bob Proctor, and David Stanley, Elvis Presley's brother.

Inspired by the transformative impact of the film "The Secret," Goldwell penned his first book, "Mastery of Abundant Living: The Keys to Mastering the Law of Attraction." He had the honor of personally presenting the first autographed copy to Bob Proctor. Recognizing that young readers may not typically engage with self-help material, Goldwell brilliantly crafted a fantastical adventure series for teens. Within these enchanting stories, he weaves principles of success and powerful life lessons to ignite hope and encourage personal growth in younger audiences.

Driven by an unwavering belief in the power of his books to change lives, Bruce Goldwell's moving journey from homeless veteran to impactful author has resonated with thousands around the globe. His triumphant quest to help others is a testament to resilience, determination, and the transformative power of words.

Dear Valued Reader,

Your thoughts and opinions matter to me,
and I kindly invite you to share your
experience by leaving a review. Your
feedback not only helps me improve our
work, but it also aids fellow readers
in discovering great stories like
this one.

I appreciate your
support and look forward to hearing
your insights!

Warm regards,
Bruce Goldwell

www.imalocalauthor.com